The Athlete's Mind

How Habit Science Enhances Performance

Benjamin H. Alexander

Table of Contents

We are what we repeatedly do. Excellence, then, is not an act, but a habit.

Chapter 1. Introduction

Immerse yourself in our exhilarating Special Report, "The Athlete's Mind: How Habit Science Enhances Performance." Discover the remarkable synergy between sports psychology and habit science, shining a light on how athletes achieve those awe-inspiring moments of glory. This riveting exploration is far from clinical jargon; it's a captivating journey into the mind of an athlete, revealing the power of habit and training in mash-up style. Don't miss out on this gripping delve into a world where mind, body, and spirit harmoniously align to push the boundaries of human potential. Ignite your own vitality and imagine new horizons in personal performance. An invigorating read awaits, offering insights you never knew you needed!

Chapter 2. The Athletic Mindset: An Introduction

Embarking on this journey of understanding, the exploration must commence from the elementary concept underpinning this stimulating report – the athletic mindset. An abstract entity, it is the amalgamation of several cognitive and emotional elements that jointly influence an athlete's performance, both during training and on the ultimate stage of competition. It is this unique mindset, a steadfast breeding ground of determination, resilience, and mental tenacity, that navigates athletes through the arduous journey 'from grassroots to glory'.

2.1. Metacognitive Elements of the Athletic Mindset

At the core of the athletic mindset are three interrelated cognitive elements: self-awareness, self-regulation, and self-efficacy. Self-awareness allows athletes to understand their strengths, weaknesses, and emotions, fostering an ever-evolving cycle of introspection and adaptation. Further, self-regulation inspires control over one's thoughts and emotions, enabling athletes to maintain composure even in high-pressure scenarios, and ensuring the consistency of their performance. Self-efficacy, on the other hand, imbues confidence in an athlete's own abilities to execute tasks, an indispensable aspect of pushing through the limitations of their comfort zones.

The athletic mindset is a proactive entity, constantly seeking improvement and adaptivity. The inclusivity of these three cognitive components, therefore, ensures that athletes approach their respective sports equipped not just with physical prowess but also a resilient mental framework primed to conquer challenges and improvise in crisis.

2.2. Emotional Intellect and the Athletic Mindset

While cognitive abilities greatly define an athlete's mindset, the role of emotional intellect cannot be undermined. The ability to perceive, understand, and manage one's emotions is a key determinant of an athlete's reaction to success, failure, and stress. A heightened sense of emotional intellect promotes resilience, helping athletes maintain stability and focus in the face of adversity.

Emotional intelligence also plays a crucial role in developing empathy, a crucial skill for team sports. It assists athletes in reading and understanding their teammates, thereby catalyzing better collaboration, fostering harmony within the team, and contributing to overall success.

2.3. Sport Specific Mindsets

Collating these traits into a defined and universal 'athletic mindset' might be simplistic due to the varied nature of sports disciplines. Factors like the type and intensity of the sport, team versus individual performance, and short versus long-duration events, govern the subtle differences in athletic mindsets. For instance, the mindset required for a marathon runner, requiring sustained endurance and solo performance, would contrast with that of a soccer player, wherein teamwork and rapid decision-making are paramount.

These subtle variations require athletes to build personalized and sport-specific mindsets, ensuring their mental and emotional framework is tailored to the unique demands of their chosen discipline. In essence, while the basic tenets of an athletic mindset remain consistent, the nuance lies in adapting them to the requirements of particular sports.

2.4. Developing the Athletic Mindset: The Role of Environment

Another fundamental though often overlooked aspect is the impact of environmental factors in shaping an athlete's mindset. Socio-cultural values, familial support, coaching style, and even peer influence play significant roles in this regard. The environment in which athletes train and grow can either encourage the cultivation of a healthy athletic mindset or unknowingly perpetuate maladaptive behaviors detrimental to their psychological well-being.

The athletic mindset, thus, is not only intrinsic but also reflective of the external influences on an athlete's life. This reciprocal relationship further adds to the complexity of understanding and developing the athletic mindset.

2.5. Athletic Mindset: The Catalyst of Habit Sciences

Given this intricate understanding of the athletic mindset, it becomes apparent that it is no mere psychological trait but a multi-faceted entity interwoven into the fabric of an athlete's daily life. This mindset becomes the driving force that nurtures habit formation, shaping the athlete's routines, rituals, and even their reaction to the challenges they face in their athletic journey.

In the forthcoming chapters, the bridging of athletic mindset with habit science will further unravel, exploring how this symbiotic relationship enhances performance, and eventually, paves the pathway to athletic glory. Our mutual exploration of this fascinating intersection of sports psychology and habit science awaits, promising to illuminate how athletes transform sheer physical exertion into awe-inspiring moments of glory.

Leaning into the athletic mindset will not only yield lucrative benefits for sportspersons but also for individuals seeking to harness the power of this mindset to bolster their resilience and determination, imbuing their lives with newfound vitality. As we delve deeper into this topic, in the chapters to come, embrace the thrill of learning with an open mind and satiate your curiosity about the remarkable mechanisms that enable peak performance in athletes. It's time to embark on this nuanced exploration of the athletic mind - a key first step in understanding how habit science can enhance performance in sports and beyond.

Chapter 3. Understanding Habit Science: The Basics

Consolidating a comprehensive understanding of habit science is the first significant stride an individual can take in unlocking a more profound comprehension of their behavior. Humans are creatures of habit, and the patterns we embody shape our world in more ways than we often realize. Before delving into this vast landscape of habit formation and its interconnection with sports performance, it's essential to begin by unfolding the rudimentary elements of this profound science.

3.1. Underpinning Foundations of Habit Science

Roles were first sung by our ancestors about how the universe was formed; patterns of stars, changing of seasons, and the rhythmic dance of life and death. The songs were their way of making sense and order from the world around them. Similarly, habits form underlying patterns in our lives, providing a predictable structure on which to hang our fleeting daily experiences.

The science of habits, or habit science, is a field that explores these patterns of behavior in people and animals. It seeks to identify the neurological, psychological, and social mechanisms that drive our actions and make us tend to repeat certain behaviors over time. However, it's important to note that habits aren't inherently negative. They are neural shortcuts—automatic behavioural responses based on learned associations—designed to promote efficiency.

3.2. The Habit Loop: Identification, Execution, Reward

At the core of habit science lies the Habit Loop, a concept popularized by Charles Duhigg in his groundbreaking book, "The Power of Habit." This model proposes that habits consist of three fundamental components: the cue, routine, and reward.

The cue is a trigger that tells the brain to initiate a particular behaviour. This could be anything from a specific location, time, preceding event, emotional state, or other associated people. The routine is the habituated action itself, executed almost subconsciously following the perception of the cue. The reward is the final part of the loop, a positive reinforcement that tells the brain that the behavior is worth remembering, further embedding it into our neural networks for future replication.

These three key elements work in unison like a well-tuned symphony orchestra, maintaining the cycle of habits.

3.3. How Habits Shape our Lives

The power of habits can't be overlooked. Habits lie so deeply ingrained in our behaviours that they shape nearly half of the decisions we make each day. Think about it; from brushing our teeth first thing in the morning to the route we drive to work or the way we tie our shoelaces - our lives are dictated more by habits than conscious decisions.

Given the extent to which they direct our actions, habits wield immense influence, shaping our health, productivity, financial security, and even interpersonal relationships to a startling degree. However, as much as habits can drive us along paths of progress and achievement, they can also anchor us in places of stagnation and harm. Being aware of our habits and learning to manipulate them to steer ourselves into advantageous pathways is a powerful tool.

3.4. The Neurology of Habits

Deep beneath the visible manifestations of our habits lies a bustling city of synaptic connections that engineer our behavioural patterns. Neural pathways, once formed, become deeply ingrained in our brains and hard to change.

As we perform an action repeatedly, the neurons involved in executing that behaviour form stronger connections, leading to synaptic plasticity. Over time, these actions require less and less conscious effort to enact, transforming into habits. Essentially, the adage 'practise makes perfect' can be rewritten more accurately as 'practice makes permanent' in the context of our neural architecture.

3.5. Habit Science: Implications and Opportunities

The understanding of habit science presents a fascinating array of implications and opportunities. Awareness of our own habit loops is the first step towards personal transformation, wherein altering an unhealthy habit or forming a new beneficial one becomes a possibility. Moreover, understanding habits can help us empathize with others, improve our relationships, and eventually, lead more fulfilled lives.

In the realm of sports performance, the importance of habit science becomes even more prominent. As we will explore in the following chapters, training isn't merely about physical ability. It's a psychological game, where understanding and manipulating habits can be the game-changer in an athlete's performance.

By gaining a nuanced understanding of habit science, we, sportspeople and non-sportspeople alike, can harness the power that habits wield, enabling us to steer our lives towards our desired goals. As we journey forward into the intertwined realms of habit science and sports performance, we will unravel even more exciting facets of this fascinating discipline, using it as a compass to navigate towards our loftiest aspirations.

Chapter 4. The Intersection of Athletics and Habit Science

As we delve into the enthralling and complex panorama of athleticism and its coalescence with the intriguing theory of habit science, it becomes imperative to understand this blend initially at a skin-deep level. Often, we marvel at an athlete's impressive performance and applaud their exceptional talent and skills. However, the concealed reality that truly fuels their power and propels them to spectacular heights is a well-articulated blend of dedicated practice, deeply ingrained habits, and a profound understanding of their capabilities, all grounded on the bedrock of habit science.

4.1. Metaphoric Unification: Athletics and Habit Science

Consider, just for a moment, athletics as an intricately woven fabric that envelopes the athlete. Habit science, then, is the intricate embroidery that accentuates the characteristic beauty of this fabric. The confluence of both these elements is an exquisite tapestry that epitomizes the athlete's superior mastery over mind and body.

Within this tapestry, athletics signifies the overt, observable actions and outcomes. They are characterized by measurable metrics such as speed, dexterity, precision, and strength. On the other hand, habit science represents the implicit, internal stimuli moulding these actions. These elements embody cognitive aspects like motivation, focus, dedication, and drive, which cannot be quantified directly but play a sine qua non role in shaping an athlete's performance.

Just as an embroidery design emerges from individual stitches woven tightly together, the application of habit science in athletics is about linking discrete actions together to form an empowering habit loop. This comprises three key elements: the cue triggering the habit, the automatic routine that follows, and the reward associated with the action. Such habit loops form the heart of an athlete's training regime, evoking consistent performance and a relentless pursuit of excellence.

4.2. Elucidating Habit Loops: The Lesser-known Champions

Appreciating the habitual context within sports requires breaking down the components of a habit loop.

The **cue**, or the trigger, is an external or internal signal prompting the brain to enact a specific routine. For athletes, these could be sights, sounds, timings, pre-game sequences, or even emotions. For instance, the whistle of a referee might be the cue for a basketball player to begin their free-throw routine.

The **routine** is the action performed in response to the cue. This is the linchpin of the habit, the specific behavior an athlete enacts without even thinking about it, thanks to repetitious training. In our example, the routine is the basketball player taking the free throw.

The **reward** is the outcome anticipated or achieved, providing the motivation to repeat the routine whenever the same cue is presented. In this case, the reward is the satisfaction of a successful free throw and the subsequent applause.

This comprehensive understanding of habit loops enables a nuanced grasp of how they serve as critical gears in the assembly line of athletic prowess. An athlete's routine can be a complex series of actions cued by sensory signals or emotional triggers, culminating in an outcome that fuels their motivation to perpetuate this cycle.

4.3. Habit Science: The Unseen Mechanic of Athletic Performance

Just as an adept mechanic goes to work under the hood of a car, improving its engine performance and longevity, habit science works behind the scenes of an athlete's consistent and precise performance. It shapes and molds cognitive processes and habitual routines, ensuring they are primed for efficient functioning.

First and foremost, understanding and awareness of habit formation reassure athletes that they aren't solely reliant on fleeting inspiration or sporadic burst of effort. Instead, they can cultivate consistent performance through ingraining certain cues and routines that lead to predictable and rewarding outcomes.

Moreover, evaluation of an athlete's existing habit loops can be invaluable in identifying performance bottlenecks and negative habits. Are there certain cues that lead to unproductive routines? Are the rewards truly motivating for the athlete? By asking these questions, players and coaches can replace unproductive elements in the habit loop and drastically elevate their performance.

Additionally, habit science also fortifies the athlete's mental resilience. Powerful habits can serve as pillars of strength during periods of stress, fatigue, or underperformance. They offer a 'default setting' to revert to when everything else might be spiraling out of control.

Furthermore, the significance of well-formed habits extends beyond the playing field, impacting athletes' lifestyle choices related to nutrition, recovery, and mental health. A better understanding of habit loops can help devise strategies to promote healthier eating, effective recovery routines, and robust mental health practices, all of which predicates superior athletic performance.

To conclude, the interface of athletics and habit science is a fascinating study, one that unveils the often imperceptible cognitive elements capably influencing an athlete's performance. It highlights that behind the spectacle of a prima donna performance on the field, there's a carefully orchestrated symphony of cues, routines, and rewards being played on the cognitive turf.

Chapter 5. Habit Formation: The Role in Sports Performance

One might claim the crux of our discourse resides in the profound interplay between habit formation and sports performance, an intricate dance that maneuvers on the tightrope of mental resilience and physical endurance. It is a relationship fraught with variables, yet intertwined with a beautiful synergy, enabling athletes to tap into the unfathomable realms of their potential.

5.1. The Anatomy of Habit: Understanding Basics

Before we delve into the enigmatic realm of habit formation, it's crucial to comprehend the basic structure of a habit. Psychology experts view habits as automated responses to specific situations developed from repetitively performing a behavior. Each habit comprises three main components—a cue, routine, and reward—often referred to as the 'habit loop.' The cue acts as a trigger, igniting the behavioral pattern (routine), followed by some form of gratification (reward), which reinforces the habit. It's an ongoing, cyclical process, subtle yet dynamic in its implications—particularly for sports performance.

5.2. Habit Formation: A Neuroscientific Perspective

The formation of habits isn't merely a psychological occurrence; it's a neuroscientific phenomenon. The Striatum, a part of the brain involved in habit formation, plays a key role in this matter. As an athlete continues repeating a task (establishing a routine), the brain gradually transitions control over to the Striatum to manage these automated functions with ease. The reason being that routines converted into habits consume less cognitive resources, allowing the brain to focus on more complex areas of athletics such as strategy and technique.

5.3. Habituation: A Pathway to Mastery

A term frequently echoed within the hallowed halls of sports psychology is habituation, the process of becoming accustomed to physically and psychologically demanding tasks. It's the essence of becoming adept at a sport. Habituation in sports is a combination of genetic potential, the surrounding environment, and targeted effort—driven by consistency and repetition, eventually leading to mastery.

By repeatedly exposing themselves to the same scenarios, athletes increase their capacity for performance, pushing their limits beyond thresholds both mentally and physically. They turn the extraordinary into the ordinary, those Herculean feats into commonplace tasks. Over time, even the most strenuous exercises become part of an athlete's comfort zone due to habitual exposure.

5.4. The Implication of Habit Formation in Sports Training

In sports training, the formation of habits plays an instrumental role. Developing the right habits leads to improved performance and achievement on the field. It's the minutiae—the tiny, well-repetitive actions, that form the cornerstone of a stellar performance.

Consider the practice schedule of a professional basketball player. It involves consistent shooting drills, cardiovascular exercises, strength training, practicing tactical plays, and reviewing match footage. Each element, when repeated and perfected, creates an automated response—a habit—that proves instrumental during competitive matches.

For a sprinter, the well-practiced routine of launching off the blocks at the sound of the starter gun is a habit ingrained into the wiring of their nervous system. In the heat of the race, there's no time for conscious thought—only the well-rehearsed response plays out. This habit formation reroutes cognitive resources toward strategies for the race ahead, securing a competitive edge.

5.5. Reforming Habits for Augmented Performance

However, the formation of habits is not exclusively beneficial. There are instances where sports athletes cultivate negative or detrimental habits, perhaps due to oversight or inappropriate training methods. The key is to unfasten these negative patterns and reform them into positive, performance-enhancing habits. It's a challenging process, yet immensely beneficial.

Integrating technologies such as biofeedback, cognitive behavioral therapy, and video analysis can contribute to detecting and rectifying these detrimental habits. Athletes can also benefit from collaborating with multidisciplinary teams, comprising coaches, trainers, sports psychologists, and nutritionists, for a comprehensive evaluation and reform of their habits.

To sum it up, habit formation, when manipulated correctly, can be a potent tool for sports performance enhancement. The key is to understand its process and mechanism, identify the habits that serve your goals, and cultivate them relentlessly, while transforming the unhelpful habits into ones that reinforce success. In the athletic world, it's not just about pushing the physical boundaries; it's about harnessing the subconscious prowess and creating habits that serve you unconsciously on the journey to immeasurable sporting triumphs.

Chapter 6. Psychological Conditioning: Techniques and Impact on Athletes

As we delve deeper into the realm of sports psychology and habit science, we reach an intriguing juncture where both disciplines firmly intersect - psychological conditioning, a fundamental pillar that underpins the success of athletes worldwide.

6.1. History and Conceptual Framework of Psychological Conditioning

Psychological conditioning is not a modern concept per se, nor exclusive to the realm of sports. It originated from the work of renowned psychologists like Ivan Pavlov and B.F. Skinner early in the 19th century. Pavlov's classical conditioning and Skinner's operant conditioning became the foundation for what we now understand as psychological conditioning, which is essentially a process that involves forming, changing, or maintaining behaviors based on the type and outcome of previous experiences.

Although originally uncovered in the general study of behavior, these theories have been meticulously applied in athletics to maximize performance. Athletes are conditioned to react in certain ways to specific stimuli, enhancing their physiological responses, psychological robustness, and ultimately, their performance on the field.

6.2. Classical Conditioning in Athletics

Remember that hungry dog in Pavlov's famous experiment? Well, it turns out that athletes aren't too dissimilar when it comes to classical conditioning. As the whistle blows, the heart races. As the starting pistol fires, muscles tense up for explosive motion. These automatic responses aren't innate but result from consistent conditioning.

Athletes are exposed to stimuli (the whistle or the pistol, for example), and over time they build a conditioned response (increased heart rate or muscle tension). It's a remarkable phenomenon, transforming what was once an indifferent stimulus into a precursor to action, enabling athletes to respond quickly and automatically, thus enhancing their performance.

6.3. Operant Conditioning in Athletics

While classical conditioning works wonders for automatic reactions, it doesn't cover all that goes into an elite athlete's performance. Enter operant conditioning — a technique that molds more complex voluntary behaviors using rewards (reinforcements) and penalties (punishments).

A football player might learn to curve the ball a certain way, rewarded by the cheer of the crowd, the satisfaction of a perfect curve, or the admiration of a coach. Conversely, a gymnast might avoid a faulty landing, having been previously penalized with deductions or the pain of injury.

This positive and negative reinforcement, or reward and punishment dynamic, can profoundly shape an athlete's behavior over time, driving exceptional performance.

6.4. The Role of Self-talk and Visualization

What about the wars waged within an athlete's mind - the self-doubt, the fear of failure? Techniques such as self-talk and visualization have been found to be essential in conditioning the mental toughness of athletes.

Self-talk is about providing reassurance, motivation, and a sense of capability to oneself, to influence one's mindset positively. A runner might repeat to himself, "I am strong. I can do this," conditioning his mind to maintain morale even under strenuous conditions.

Similarly, visualization involves athletes imagining themselves performing specific tasks successfully. By doing so, they condition their minds to anticipate success, creating a positive ripple effect that extends to their actual performance.

6.5. Techniques in Action: Case Studies

Consider the famous basketball player – Michael Jordan. Despite being naturally gifted, Jordan practiced intensely, often repeating shots and plays until they were perfect. He used both forms of conditioning: the sounds of the court (classical), the satisfaction of successful shots (operant), and drained three-pointers themselves became stimuli that prompted excellence.

On the other hand, we have elite swimmer Michael Phelps who is known to visualize his perfect race every night before sleep. He conditions his mind to aim for perfect strokes, turns, and finishes, reinforcing his mental toughness and performance.

6.6. Psychological Conditioning: A Synergy between Mind and Body

Ultimately, psychological conditioning is about achieving an exceptional symbiosis between the athlete's mind and the robustness of their physique. It's about making the body react effectively to the mind's signals, as well as aligning the mind to accomplish its tasks despite external pressure.

Both the mind and body of an athlete are subject to conditioning through stimuli, rewards, and punishments, and effective psychological conditioning lies in balancing these elements.

As we continue to explore the intersection of sports psychology and habit science, it becomes more evident that the success of athletes isn't merely a measure of physical prowess, but also a testament to their mental fortitude and discipline, achieved through positive conditioning. New avenues are always emerging in this fascinating interplay between mind and body, paving the way for future athletes to push the boundaries of human performance even further.

Chapter 7. The Power of Rituals and Routines in Sports

In a thrilling expedition into the world of sport, the role of rituals and routines emerges as a key factor that aids athletes in the constant pursuit of performance enhancement. While physical prowess and natural talent are often noted as cornerstones of athletic success, delving deeper into the subject uncovers the power of habitual patterns that define an athlete's rhythm: their rituals and routines.

7.1. The Essence of Rituals and Routines in Sports

Rituals and routines in sports are systematic and, often, symbolic procedures carried out by athletes prior to, during, or after their performance. These routines lend a sense of familiarity and control amidst various uncontrollable variables that characterize the world of sports.

Structured and repetitive actions or thoughts form the bedrock of these rituals, providing the athlete with a sense of grounding and focus that is vital for maintaining composure and gearing up for the task at hand. The process of habituation plays a critical role in instilling these routines within an athlete's regimen. Over time, these actions become second nature, providing an undercurrent of stability and constancy amidst the dynamic sport environment.

7.2. Understanding the Difference: Rituals Versus Routines

To fully grasp the nature of rituals and routines in sport, it's crucial to differentiate between these two terms. While both entail a series of actions performed predictably and consistently, it's the underlying psyche that demarcates them. Routines are essentially goal-directed and functional activities carried out methodically in a certain order. They are based on rational grounds and have an explicit objective in relation to athletic performance - for instance, a warm-up routine before practicing on the field.

Rituals, on the other hand, generally involve symbolic and superstitious beliefs with no concrete 'cause-effect' relationship to the sport performance. They are traditionally associated with producing a state of mental preparation and positive mindset, even if the actions might seem illogical or unnecessary from the functional perspective. Athletes have been known to wear 'lucky' shoes, touch a particular object, or carry out a string of actions 'just-so' based on personal or cultural belief systems.

Despite their differences, both rituals and routines have equally transformative potential when it comes to athlete's mental conditioning and performance.

7.3. The Psychological Catalysts: Familiarity and Focus

What role do rituals and routines play in shaping the mind of an athlete? The answer to this question lies in the psychological comfort lent by familiarity and focus.

Rituals and routines form a sort of- 'psychological home', a safe mental space that athletes can access amidst performance-related stress. Over time, these patterns become familiar - a predictable element in an unpredictable environment. Such consistency often provides a sense of comfort, instills self-confidence, and reduces performance anxiety. Often, these routines also serve as psychological triggers that help athletes transition into their performance 'zone'.

Moreover, these systematic processes demand focus, harnessing the athlete's attention towards a specific series of tasks. This directed attention provides a mental warm-up and encourages mindfulness, which in turn helps to enhance concentration levels during the sports performance.

7.4. Sports Rituals and Routines: Case Study

To observe the application of these customary workings, we can turn to Serena Williams, the queen of the tennis court. Known for her powerful strokes, Serena also highlights the understated power of rituals and routines in sports. From bouncing the ball exactly five times before her first serve to wearing the same pair of socks throughout the tournament for good luck, Serena's sporting journey is punctuated with these repetitive actions. They serve not only as mental primers but also add a rhythmic quality to her performance, helping her bring her best game to every match.

The final point worth underscoring is the dynamic nature of these rituals and routines. They can evolve with the athlete, changing and adapting to new environments, pressures, and demands of the sport - marking the ongoing dialogue between habit science and athletic performance.

As we pull back from this comprehensive exploration, the significance of these habits becomes even more stark. Rituals and routines remain a cornerstone in the athletic world, allowing athletes to harness control and familiarity into their performances – creating a harmony of body and mind that complements their physical endeavors.

In the subsequent chapters, we will continue our exploration of these fascinating habits and analyze more case studies that illuminate their value in enhancing sports performance, overcoming challenges, and transforming athletic potential.

Chapter 8. Case Studies: Successful Athletes and Their Habits

The riveting tales of athletes who have achieved extraordinary feats often overshadow the hard work, sacrifice, and tenacity that propels them to such heights. It's not solely innate talent or physical prowess that take athletes to such levels of achievement, it's the habits they cultivate. These habits play a crucial role, shaping their preparation and performance.

8.1. The Art Of Practice: Michael Jordan

Michael Jordan, arguably the greatest basketball player ever, was not naturally gifted at the sport. In fact, he was rejected from his high school team the first time. However, he did not allow this setback to deter him. Instead, Jordan began to practice relentlessly.

His commitment to practice became ingrained as a habit, leading to the development of an exceptional skill set. Jordan once said, "I've always believed that if you put in the work, the results will come." But it wasn't just about the time spent on the court, it was also about the quality of his practice. Jordan didn't just practice, he practiced with intention, always trying to improve specific weak points in his game. He also made it a point to practice under pressure to simulate real game situations.

8.2. Persistence Against All Odds: Serena Williams

Serena Williams' career is a prime example of of habit-driven success. The routine she developed from a young age, instilled by her father Richard, not only consisted of gruelling physical training, but also incorporated a mental toughness regimen.

This ethos of 'never give up', a habit she absorbed, has consistently played a tremendous role in her career. This has been obviously apparent in numerous matches, where she has successfully rallied from seemingly insurmountable positions to clinch victory. Williams' insurmountable resolve, her refusal to surrender, typifies a habit of persistence that pervades her career.

8.3. The Detailed Regimen: Cristiano Ronaldo

Cristiano Ronaldo stands as a paragon of meticulous discipline. His thorough training regimen is a testament to his commitment to the sport and talent. His day begins and ends early, with meticulously planned meals, finely-tuned workouts, routine recovery sessions, and even specific sleeping schedules.

Ronaldo's habits extend beyond fitness and diet. He implements strategies like visualization, a technique where an athlete imagines themselves succeeding and scoring. Ronaldo has adopted these habits to augment his performance, providing him a holistic approach to his career that enables his phenomenal success on the field.

8.4. Mastering The Mind: Michael Phelps

Michael Phelps, the most decorated Olympian of all time, has long championed the power of mental preparation in sports. Beyond his rigorous physical training, Phelps relied heavily on visualization techniques, literally picturing his races and victories in his mind before they happened.

Phelps' coach, Bob Bowman, helped him develop this habit, which Phelps refined over time thoroughly visualizing each race, each stroke, even the sensation of water on his skin. This routine helped eradicate fear and doubt from Phelps' mind, and filled him with an unwavering belief in his ability to win.

In conclusion, it becomes apparent that habits, the conscious repetition of actions that eventually become second nature, play an integral role in the success narrative of an athlete. These routines, ingrained into their daily lives, accumulating over time, have a profound impact on their performance. Painstaking practice, dogged determination, stringent self-discipline and meticulous mental preparation - the story of each athlete testified to the power of these habits. Each case illustrates that the road to glory is not only about the destination, it's also about the journey, habit by habit, step by step. Every rigorous training session, every disciplined approach to nutrition, every visualisation technique serves its time in the athletics' narrative to form an impregnable fortitude for commanding performance on international stages.

Chapter 9. Transforming Performance: Applying Habits in Everyday Training

The concept of habit formation and retention doesn't exist in void. It captures its true essence when it's applied in real life scenarios, and for an athlete, those scenarios often revolve around their everyday training regimes. In the context of athletics, the habits of an athlete extend way beyond the scope of their respective sports. They form an integral part of an athlete's lifestyle and have a profound impact on their performance. One must understand that excellence in sports doesn't simply hinge on a few peak moments of exceptional performance during a match or a competition, but rather, it's the result of consistent, relentless training framed by healthy habits and mental conditioning.

9.1. Understanding the Significance of Habits in Training

To appreciate the importance of habits in training, it might be helpful to look at the process of getting better in a sport as a loop. This loop starts with learning, moves through practicing, and finally ends at performing. Learning happens when an athlete acquires new skills; practicing happens when these skills are repeated over and over again, and performance happens when these practiced skills are executed in a real competitive scenario. Now, where do habits fit in this loop? They're all pervasive. Habits make the process of learning faster, the process of practicing more effective, and the process of performing more consistent.

Each of these processes can be thought of as a path through a jungle. The first time an athlete learns a new skill, they are essentially hacking their way through dense vegetation. Practice then becomes a way to tread that same path again and again until it's a well-worn trail - easy to follow without significant conscious thought, making the behavior almost automatic. Essentially, habits transform the new skill into a well-beaten path.

9.2. Forming Performance-enhancing Habits

An athlete's habits play a significant role in determining their performance. Thus, it is imperative to form result-oriented habits that have a positive impact on training outcomes. To this end, the science of habit formation is based on a three-step process - the cue, the routine, and the reward.

The Cue: It is the trigger that initiates the habit. For instance, an athlete may have the cue of lacing up their running shoes early in the morning. This seemingly simple action primes their mind for the routine to follow.

The Routine: This is the actual habituated behavior. In our example, it might be going for a run, performing a set of stretches, or following a specific dietary schedule.

The Reward: This is the outcome that positively reinforces the routine, making the habit more likely to be repeated. In the context of training, this could be the feeling of satisfaction post a strenuous workout, the sense of accomplishment after another personal best has been broken, or even the physical benefits brought by these routines.

Knowing and applying this framework of habit formation is instrumental for athletes looking to form training-related habits. This understanding allows them to identify the cues that lead to desired routines and the rewards that reinforce them.

9.3. Overcoming Inertia and Resisting Laziness

Perhaps the biggest hurdle in the path of habit formation is the inertia of comfort and the allure of laziness. This inertia can be a formidable enemy, more so in the context of training, where the routines involve significant physical exertion.

An effective approach to overcoming inertia is by starting small - the initial aim should be just to start. One shouldn't worry too much about the time duration of the training or its intensity in initial stages. The first step could be as simple as getting up at a certain time or getting dressed for the workout. Breaking an entire process down into smaller, more manageable tasks can help an athlete ease into a new system until the entire process eventually becomes habitual.

Likewise, resisting laziness often involves mind games. Visual reminders like setting out the training gear the night before or daily motivational charts can serve as both cues and motivators. These visual cues alleviate laziness by reminding the athlete about their long term goals and immediate tasks.

9.4. Habit Stacking: A Powerful Tool

A useful technique often followed by athletes in habit formation is habit stacking. This involves tying a new habit to an already existing one. An existing habit essentially serves as the cue for the new routine, thus making habit formation easier. For example, an athlete could attach the act of meditation immediately after their daily regimen of warm-up exercises. Here, the completion of the warm-up exercise acts as the cue for the meditation habit.

9.5. Case Study: The Famous Swimmer's Routine

Consider the example of Michael Phelps, the most decorated Olympian ever, to understand the integration of these concept. His coach, Bob Bowman, meticulously engineered a specific routine to prime Phelps for prime performance. It started with playing a mixtape that Phelps had listened to before every major victory in his room; this served as the cue. The actual routine comprised of a regimented series of activities starting with stretching, then swimming for a precisely determined duration at an exact pace, and finally cooling down. The reward was the sense of complete preparation and focused readiness. This routine so deeply ingrained in Phelps that it ran almost autonomically, driving him to unprecedented records and victories.

9.6. In Closing: The Long Journey Ahead

Applying habits in everyday training is a long, meticulous, and sometimes grueling process. It involves hours of conscious effort, understanding the mechanics of one's own mindset, and an unswerving dedication towards the cause.

Nonetheless, it is a journey worth embarking upon. Transforming one's performance through habituated training routines not only augments the potential for success in competitive scenarios, but it also infuses an athlete's daily life with a sense of purpose, discipline, balance, and ultimately, the satisfaction that comes from reaching their potential in their chosen field. Emboldening these practices will undeniably foster a mindset that strives for growth, promoting the athlete's progression even beyond the realm of sports.

Chapter 10. Tackling Challenges: Overcoming Bad Habits in Sports

In the world of sports, one might be led to believe that performance improvement is an inevitable gradual progression, following hours, weeks, even years of intense training. However, what is less often spoken about - but no less critical in the path to athletes' greatness - are those habitual behavioral grooves, deep and tricky to navigate, rightly termed as 'bad habits.' These habits remain stubborn obstacles that, if not properly tackled, can significantly hinder an athlete's breakthrough performance.

10.1. Identification of Bad Habits

The battle with unwanted habits is a quest that starts with identification. Recognizing the difference between good and bad habits is paramount. Bad routines in sports can be physical, like improper form or technique, or they can be mental, such as negative self-talk or excessive performance anxiety. In order to identify these, it is essential to observe an athlete's performance closely, whether through video analysis, feedback from coaches, or self-reflection.

Athletes may also take advantage of various technological tools, which are increasingly becoming instrumental in tracking and assessing performance. Sophisticated performance analysis software and biometric wearable technology are among the advancements responsible for augmenting our understanding of sports metrics, and subsequently, they are proving crucial in the process of habit identification.

10.2. Techniques for Overcoming Bad Habits

Once identified, the true toiling begins – eradicating these habits involves a combination of relentless effort, sound strategies, and continual perseverance. One prominent method is leveraging 'habit replacement,' essentially replacing a bad habit with a more beneficial one.

For instance, consider an athlete struggling with poor nutrition due to the habit of consuming fast food. They can progressively replace this habit with healthier eating behaviors, initially by swapping one meal a day. Gradually this act becomes automatic, replacing the previous detrimental habit.

Contrary to perceived assumptions, 'abrupt cessation,' entirely eliminating an undesirable habit suddenly, often proves counterproductive. This method can lead to psychological stress and potential relapse, thus gentle, gradual changes are often more effective long-term solutions.

Cognitive behavioral therapy (CBT) is another proven technique. Athletes can employ CBT to challenge negative thought patterns and unhealthy behaviors, developing healthier, more positive cognitive habits instead. Similarly 'exposure therapy,' systematically and progressively facing the situation or behavior you want to change, can facilitate habit reconstruction.

But, undeniably, consistency is key. As Aristotle once said, "We are what we repeatedly do. Excellence, then, is not an act but a habit."

10.3. Role of a Support System

The role of a robust support system in overcoming bad habits cannot be underestimated. Support systems can take many forms - coaches, mentors, teammates, family, or friends - and the contribution of these individuals is pivotal. They can offer much-needed emotional support, objective feedback, and a sense of accountability, reinforcing an athlete's commitment to shattering unfavorable habits.

10.4. Habit Tracking and Maintenance

Maintaining the eradication of bad habits is an ongoing task. It requires a lifelong commitment and requires effective tracking systems. This is where habit trackers come in. Habit tracking is the practice of recording every instance of a habit, beneficial or detrimental. From simple tick mark systems to complex habit tracking apps, these tools offer a visual representation of progress, which can be incredibly motivating in the pursuit of excellence.

Moreover, as well as being a method of reward, tracking also offers an opportunity for course correction. Regular monitoring can reveal if an athlete is relapsing, allowing proactive steps to avoid slipping back into old, detrimental ways.

10.5. Conclusion

Overcoming bad habits in sports, though indeed a challenging proposition, shapes a critical step towards athletic excellence. It is a process of constant diligence, of probing for those imperfections lurking beneath the surface of an athlete's performance, and diligently rooting them out. With the right identification techniques, the application of proven coping strategies, a supportive environment, and robust tracking systems, athletes can transform their destructive habits into constructions ones, touching new pinnacles of performance, pushing the boundaries of human potential.

Chapter 11. Future of Sports: The Expanding Role of Habit Science

Our exciting journey ends on the promising horizon of the future, where we glimpse into the expanding potential of habit science in the realm of sports. Unarguably, there is a rising interest and understanding of the immense power that habits hold over our actions and consequently, our sporting performances. As we step forward in the labyrinth of time, it is the amalgamation of sports psychology and habit science that waves a promising future filled with bountiful opportunities and advancements.

11.1. The Current Evolution of Habit Science in Sports

Habit science began as a vague concept trying to understand the mystical workings of psyche, behavior, and performances. It has now flourished into a diverse, interdisciplinary field, offering its valuable insights to sports for the enhancement of athletes' routines and performances. This evolution is rooted in the intersection of technology, neuroscience, and psychology. The technological advancements have allowed us to delve deeper into the brain's intricate workings, unveiling the neurobiological foundations of habits.

The discipline of neuroscience effectively maps the brain changes during habit formation, reflecting the neuroplasticity that fosters motor skills and cognitive routines. These insights have opened new avenues for sports training, accentuating the significance of repetitive practice and mental conditioning to reinforce neural pathways. In parallel, psychology elucidates the motivational and cognitive processes underlining habit formation. These concurrent developments in neuroscience and psychology lay down the road for the current evolution of habit science from a holistic perspective.

11.2. Looking Forward: Predicting Future Developments

Image Caption: A conceptual image showcasing the future intersection of sport, neuroscience, and psychology

The future of habit science within sports suggests a more personalized and comprehensive approach to athlete training. As data-driven decision-making becomes paramount, habit science will likely introduce innovative ways to create individualized training routines.

Furthermore, the continuous interaction between habit science, coaching, and talent development professionals will advance evidence-based interventions. These planned interventions can promote positive habit formation while mitigating detrimental habits. The application of habit science is not limited to athletic performances alone. We foresee its tremendous potential in shaping the athlete's life outside the world of sports.

11.3. Building Sports Ecosystems that Foster Healthy Habits

An essential part of the future application of habit science lies not only in the hand of athletes or coaches but in establishing entire sports ecosystems that cultivate healthy habits. By embedding habit science-infused practices into sports environments, we can ensure that the influence of habit formation extends far beyond the training ground.

Habit-friendly sports environments will likely focus on incorporating mental conditioning alongside physical training, promoting a culture of well-being, emphasizing on positive reinforcements, and offering support systems that cater to the holistic development of athletes.

11.4. The Interdisciplinary Approach: Bridging Gaps

Habit science, being interdisciplinary, is characterized by the convergence of multiple disciplines, holding the potential to bridge the gaps among various sporting domains. This multidisciplinary integration is expected to revolutionize the way athletes train, perform, recover, and maintain their psychological well-being.

The path forward involves further cooperation among sports psychologists, neuroscientists, and coaches who can cohesively work towards the common goal of refining athlete performance through data-backed habit interventions.

11.5. Summary

Our peek into the future of sports and the role of habit science tells a tale of immense potential. We stand at the cusp of a promising future where habit science will play a crucial role in shaping athletic performance, providing a framework for focused, targeted, and efficient training methods. This shift towards habit-oriented sports will foster healthier athletes, imbue a sense of holistic well-being within sports ecosystems, and potentially alter the sports landscape as we know it.

Indeed, the future of sports is habit-infused, and we are only beginning to tap into this exciting new frontier. Emboldened by advancements in neuroscience, technology, and psychology, habit science is opening new avenues for growth, development, and unparalleled achievements within the sphere of athletics. Herein lies the true essence of the expanding role of habit science within sports - a gateway to a future where mind, body, and spirit harmonize in the pursuit of excellence.

www.ingramcontent.com/pod-product-compliance
Lightning Source LLC
Chambersburg PA
CBHW061534250726
48657CB00005B/2226